Title: Hope beyond the diagnosis: Finding a new normal with Kidney failure.

stephanie c. Reaves

INTRODUCTION

The diagnosis that changes everything

A diagnosis is a defining moment in life. It has the power to upend the very fabric of our reality and change the path of our life in ways we never could have anticipated. The diagnosis that alters everything causes a significant alteration in how we view ourselves, our lives, and our futures rather than just being a medical proclamation. The diagnosis that alters everything, whether it be a fatal illness, a terrible accident, or a chronic sickness, is a defining event that can be both devastating and transforming.

When we receive a diagnosis, we are forced to face the fact that we are not immortal and that things could not turn out the way we expect them to. We are made to face our own mortality and the transience of life. It is normal to experience a variety of feelings, such as fear, anger, despair, and disbelief, in response to this discovery, which can be overpowering.

A diagnosis that completely alters a person's life can leave them feeling profoundly lost. We lament losing our health, our freedom, and our aspirations for the future.

We can feel that the person we were before the diagnosis has changed. We could find it difficult to adjust to this new reality because the world can appear to be a frightening and unsettling place.

A life-altering diagnosis, though, can also serve as a springboard for development and change on a personal level. It might make us confront the issues that actually matter in life and establish priorities. We can discover that we have a fresh appreciation for the people and things that make us happy and fulfilled. We might find a courage and fortitude we didn't know we have.

Uncertainty is one of the most difficult aspects of receiving a diagnosis that completely alters your life. It can be really frightening to not know what the future holds. But it's crucial to keep in mind that we're not the only ones going through this. We have resources and people at our disposal to help us on our path.

Putting our attention on the things we can control can help us deal with the uncertainty of a diagnosis. This can entail altering one's way of life by switching to a better diet, increasing one's physical activity, and lowering one's stress levels. It might also entail asking friends, family, and medical experts for assistance. Having a solid support system might be crucial for overcoming the difficulties that come with a diagnosis.

Taking care of our mental health is a crucial part of adjusting to a diagnosis that fundamentally alters our lives. A variety of emotions are normal to feel, and it's crucial to recognise and express them in a healthy way. This can be speaking with a therapist or counselor, keeping a journal, or doing something artistic or musically creative.

It is crucial to advocate for both ourselves and other people in addition to looking after our own mental health. This could entail learning more about our disease and available treatments, getting second opinions, and joining support groups and advocacy groups. We can assist create awareness and encourage constructive change by speaking up and sharing our experiences.

It's not easy to receive a diagnosis that alters everything, but it may be a life-changing event that fosters development, resiliency, and hope. It might be necessary for us to give up our old habits and accept a new standard of living. To find new methods to give our life meaning and purpose, we may need to rethink what happiness and success mean to us.

In the end, the diagnosis that alters everything can present an opportunity to consider what is truly important in life and to live more deliberately and purposefully. It may serve as a reminder of how valuable life is and how each moment is a gift. We can find hope and significance in the midst of difficulty by accepting the difficulties and uncertainties that come with a diagnosis.

The search for hope

One of the fundamental aspects of the human experience is the desire for hope. We set out on this search when we are feeling uncertain, afraid, or doubtful. Whether we are dealing with a personal catastrophe, a worldwide pandemic, or a significant shift in our lives, hope is the light that leads us through the night and motivates us to keep going.

Hope is fundamentally the conviction that things will improve. It is a feeling of hope and assurance that the future is full with potential. Hope is a firm belief in our capacity to overcome adversity and build a better society, not naive optimism or wishful thinking.

There are numerous ways to look for hope. It might entail looking for sources of inspiration in literature, music, or the arts. It could entail looking to spirituality or religion for direction and solace. It can entail asking friends, family, or medical experts for assistance.

Building resiliency is one of the most crucial components of the search for hope. Resilience is the capacity to overcome adversity, adjust to novel situations, and flourish in the face of difficulty. We can learn to be resilient over time; it's not a quality that comes naturally to us.

There are numerous approaches to building resilience. One strategy is to concentrate on the variables under our control. This could entail making minor adjustments to our daily routine, like exercising more, cultivating mindfulness, or scheduling time for self-care. It might also entail changing the way we think about difficulties and failures so that we see them as chances for development and education rather than as insurmountable obstacles.

Creating a solid support system is another crucial component in developing resilience. This can entail asking friends, relatives, or medical experts for assistance. It might also entail getting in touch with people who have experienced similar things, such joining a support group or advocacy group.

The pursuit of hope might also entail learning to be grateful and appreciative of the present. It can be simple to concentrate on the things we don't have or the difficulties we are experiencing, but by focusing on the things we do have, we can develop a sense of thankfulness and contentment.

Connection is one of the most potent sources of hope. Being connected to others, to nature, and to something more than ourselves may be a great source of comfort and inspiration. Connection can give us a sense of purpose and belonging, whether it be through volunteering, spending time in nature, or engaging in spiritual activities.

The quest for hope is ultimately a trip we must take on for ourselves. On this path, we must be open to the prospect of a better future and honest with ourselves about our worries and uncertainties. It challenges us to practice resilience, thankfulness, and connection while maintaining hope that things will improve.

The hunt for optimism might occasionally seem overpowering and unachievable. We could feel as though we are sinking beneath a sea of hopelessness and uncertainty. However, it is at these times when hope is most crucial. The light of hope is strongest when things are at their darkest; it acts as a beacon, guiding us out of the shadows and into a better future.

It is simple to lose sight of the things that give us hope when we are faced with adversity. We can believe that we are in a hopeless situation, that no one knows what we are going through, or that we are all alone. We must always keep in mind that we are never truly alone. Even in the most difficult times, there are people and things that can help us.

The pursuit of hope is a lifelong journey rather than a singular event. It is a path that calls for us to never give up, to grow resilience and gratitude, and to be open to new experience.

CHAPTER 1:

NAVIGATING THE DIAGNOSIS

Understanding kidney failure:what it means and what to expect

A condition known as kidney failure, often referred to as renal failure, occurs when the kidneys are unable to adequately filter waste and extra fluid from the circulation. As a result, toxins may accumulate in the body, which may result in a number of symptoms and problems.

Kidney failure comes in two flavors: acute and chronic. An accident, an infection, or a medicine are just a few examples of the many things that can lead to acute renal failure, which is a sudden loss of kidney function. On the other hand, chronic kidney failure is a decrease of kidney function that happens gradually over months or years.

The signs of renal failure can be identical in both situations. The following are some typical signs of renal failure:

•Changes in urine flow, including decreased output or increased frequency of urination •Fatigue •Swelling in the legs and ankles •Shortness of breath •Nausea and vomiting •Loss of appetite
People with kidney failure may also face problems like high blood pressure, anemia, bone disease, and fluid accumulation in the lungs in addition to these symptoms.

A combination of blood and urine tests, as well as imaging tests like CT or ultrasound scans, are frequently used to diagnose kidney failure. The underlying cause of renal failure and the severity of the symptoms will determine the best course of treatment.

The management of the underlying cause of the ailment, such as stopping a medication that might be harming the kidneys or curing an infection, may be used to treat acute renal failure. To eliminate extra fluid and waste from the blood, dialysis may occasionally be required.

Treatment options for chronic kidney failure may include a mix of prescription drugs, dietary adjustments, and dialysis or kidney transplantation. To assist control symptoms and stop the disease's progression, doctors may prescribe medications. A low-salt diet and frequent exercise can assist improve kidney function, among other lifestyle modifications.

People with chronic renal failure may occasionally have the option of a kidney transplant. A healthy kidney from a donor is surgically transplanted into the body of the recipient during a kidney transplant. Although a kidney transplant can be a highly effective treatment for renal disease, it carries some risks and needs constant monitoring and care.

Living with renal failure can be difficult on a physical and psychological level. People who have kidney failure might need to make significant dietary and lifestyle adjustments and could need ongoing medical attention and support. To control symptoms and create a treatment plan that is tailored to each patient's needs, it is crucial to work closely with a healthcare team.

People with renal failure may benefit from psychological and emotional support in addition to medical care. Managing the emotional and practical issues of renal failure requires having a support system in place because dealing with a chronic illness may be stressful and exhausting.

Among some suggestions for treating renal failure are:

•Eating a low-salt, low-fat diet to control blood pressure and ease renal strain
•Regular exercise, under the direction of a medical professional, to support symptom management and general health maintenance.
•Manage drugs with caution, taking them as directed and keeping an eye out for any potential adverse effects.
•Reaching out to loved ones, friends, support groups, or medical professionals for emotional and psychological assistance.
•Keeping up-to-date on the ailment and available therapies, as well as collaborating closely with a medical team to create a tailored treatment strategy.
Although having kidney failure might be difficult, it's vital to keep in mind that there are treatments available

to control symptoms and enhance quality of life. People with kidney failure can live full and meaningful lives by collaborating closely with a healthcare team, modifying their lifestyles, and enlisting the assistance of friends, family, and healthcare professionals.

Coping with the diagnosis: Tips for emotional and mental wellbeing.

Being told that you have a chronic condition can be frightening and stressful. It can be challenging to manage the mental and physical difficulties that come with a chronic illness, so it's crucial to give attention to emotional and mental wellbeing as part of an all-encompassing treatment plan.

Here are some pointers for managing a diagnosis of a chronic illness and preserving emotional and mental health:

1. Recognize your feelings: After receiving a diagnosis of a chronic illness, it's common to feel a variety of emotions, such as fear, anger, grief, and frustration.

Instead of attempting to repress or ignore these emotions, it is critical to identify and validate them. To help you process and manage these emotions, consider talking to a close friend or family member or thinking about getting professional support.

2. Educate yourself: Knowing more about the illness might help you feel more in control and less anxious. Spend some time learning about the illness, its signs and symptoms, and the potential therapies. Request information and resources from your medical team, and think about joining support groups or online discussion forums to meet people who are dealing with the same disease.

3. Establish reasonable goals. A chronic illness can result in several lifestyle modifications and restrictions, so it's crucial to establish realistic goals for what you can do. Concentrate on short-term objectives that are doable, like picking up a new pastime or adding light exercise to your daily routine. No matter how minor they may seem, acknowledge and celebrate these successes.

4. Take care of yourself: Self-care is an important part of treating a chronic condition. This can involve things like

getting enough rest, maintaining a balanced diet, and practicing stress-relieving exercises like yoga or meditation. Self-care must be given top priority as part of an all-encompassing therapeutic strategy.

5. Keep in touch: Having a chronic illness can make you feel isolated, but it's crucial to keep in touch with other people. Call on your friends and family for help, or think about signing up for online forums or support groups to meet people who are experiencing the same thing. To keep a sense of connection and purpose, think about volunteering or taking part in activities that you find interesting.

6. Use stress-reduction strategies: treating stress is a crucial component of treating a chronic condition. Think about introducing stress-relieving practices like progressive muscle relaxation, visualization, or deep breathing into your everyday routine. These methods can lessen anxiety and enhance general wellbeing.

7. Seek professional assistance: If you are finding it difficult to handle a diagnosis of a chronic illness, it is crucial to seek expert assistance. Working with a

therapist or counselor, joining a support group, or using an internet forum are a few examples of how to do this. Your medical staff can also suggest services and contacts for assistance with your mental health.

8. Adopt a positive outlook: A positive outlook can be a useful management technique for a chronic condition. Instead of concentrating on what you can't do, try to think about what you can. Celebrate modest successes and cultivate gratitude for the positive aspects of your life.

9. Keep an open line of communication with your medical team: Throughout the duration of your illness, it's crucial to keep an open line of communication with your medical team. By doing so, you may make sure that you are receiving the right care and attention, as well as help identify any early-stage difficulties or side effects.

10. Speak out for yourself: You have the right to actively participate in your own care as a patient. Ask questions, voice concerns, and, if need, get second perspectives as you represent yourself. Keep up-to-date on your disease

and available treatments, and collaborate with your healthcare team to create an extensive treatment plan.

Even though managing a chronic illness might be difficult, a thorough treatment plan should put a high priority on one's mental and emotional health. Individuals can handle the emotional and mental problems that come with a chronic illness diagnosis and lead fulfilling lives by engaging in self-care, maintaining relationships with others, and obtaining professional support when necessary.

Treatment options: Dialysis, Transplantation and other approaches.

End-stage renal disease (ESRD), often known as kidney failure, is a significant medical illness that develops when the kidneys can no longer function normally. Kidney failure can be treated in a variety of ways, including dialysis, transplantation, and other methods. The many kidney failure treatment options, as well as their advantages and disadvantages, will be covered in this article.

•Dialysis:

When the kidneys are unable to filter waste and extra fluid from the blood, a medical procedure called dialysis is used. Hemodialysis and peritoneal dialysis are the two basic forms of dialysis.

•Hemodialysis:

Hemodialysis is a type of dialysis in which the blood is filtered through an artificial kidney, or dialyzer. Hemodialysis involves removing blood from the body, pumping it through a dialyzer to filter out waste and extra fluid, and then reintroducing the blood to the body. Hemodialysis normally takes place in a hospital or dialysis facility and lasts for many hours each time. It is commonly done three times per week.

Dialysis in the peritoneum

The peritoneum, or lining of the abdomen, is used to filter blood during peritoneal dialysis. Through a tiny catheter, a particular fluid is injected into the abdomen during peritoneal dialysis and remains there for several hours. Before being drained from the body, the fluid draws waste and extra fluid from the blood. Home peritoneal dialysis is an option, and it is frequently performed daily and more frequently than hemodialysis.

Dialysis's advantages and disadvantages

Dialysis is a successful treatment for renal failure that prolongs life and improves quality of life for patients. Dialysis does have a few downsides, though. Dialysis takes time and can be emotionally and physically taxing. It also calls for stringent adherence to hydration and nutritional limitations, which can be challenging to handle. Additionally, patients must continue receiving therapy for the remainder of their lives because dialysis does not treat renal failure.

•Transplantation:

A healthy kidney from a living or deceased donor is surgically placed into a patient with renal failure during a kidney transplant. As it gives a patient a functioning kidney and enables them to lead a somewhat normal life, kidney transplantation is the most successful treatment for renal failure. However, kidney transplantation is not without its difficulties.

Donor scarcity

The lack of available organs is one of the main issues with kidney transplantation. In the United States alone, there are currently over 100,000 persons on the kidney transplant waiting list, and there is a severe shortage of kidneys. As a result, patients now have to wait a very long time for kidney transplants, and many of them pass away in the process.

Transplant rejection

The possibility of transplant rejection is another difficulty connected with kidney transplantation.

Transplant rejection, which can cause the transplanted kidney to fail, happens when the body's immune system assaults the donated kidney as a foreign item. Patients must take immunosuppressive drugs for the remainder of their lives to prevent transplant rejection, which can have negative side effects.

Other strategies

There are numerous different methods of treating renal failure outside dialysis and transplantation, including:

•Conservative leadership:

An alternative to harsh medical measures, conservative care focuses on treating symptoms and enhancing quality of life. Patients with multiple comorbidities, advanced age, or other conditions that render them unsuitable for dialysis or transplantation may benefit from this method.

•Medical management: includes controlling symptoms and complications in addition to addressing the underlying cause of kidney failure. Patients with mild to moderate kidney failure or patients who are not strong candidates for dialysis or transplantation due to other medical issues may benefit from this method. Medical care may involve prescription drugs to lower cholesterol and blood pressure as well as lifestyle changes like dietary adjustments and frequent exercise.

Alternative therapies: have been investigated as potential treatments for kidney failure. Examples include acupuncture, herbal remedies, and massage therapy. While there is no evidence that these therapies will cure renal failure, some people may find them useful for controlling symptoms like pain and anxiety.

Clinical studies:

Clinical trials are research projects that evaluate potential renal failure treatments. Clinical trial participants gain access to cutting-edge remedies and may aid in the creation of fresh renal failure treatments.

In summary, there are numerous ways to treat renal failure, including dialysis, transplantation, and other methods. Every treatment method has advantages and disadvantages, and the best course of action will be determined by the patient's age, general health, and personal preferences. Patients with kidney failure should consult closely with their medical team to choose the best course of action for their unique need. Despite the fact that kidney failure is a serious medical illness, people can have happy and rewarding lives with the correct care and support.

CHAPTER 2:

FINDING YOUR NEW NORMAL

Lifestyle changes: managing your diet,exercise and medication

Modifying one's lifestyle is crucial for controlling renal failure. Lifestyle changes can help delay the progression of the disease and enhance general health and wellbeing in addition to medical treatments like dialysis and transplantation. In this section, we'll talk about how to properly manage renal failure by controlling your food, exercise routine, and medicine.

1. Keeping a Dietary Plan:

Managing one's food is one of the most crucial lifestyle adjustments for kidney failure sufferers. This is because certain foods and beverages can exacerbate renal impairment since the kidneys are in charge of filtering waste and extra fluid from the body. It's common practice to counsel renal failure patients to restrict their intake of particular foods and beverages, such as:

•**Sodium**: Too much sodium can lead to fluid retention and high blood pressure, both of which worsen kidney disease. Patients with renal disease are frequently told to keep their daily salt consumption under 2,300 milligrams.

•**Potassium**: Excess potassium in the blood can accumulate when the kidneys are not functioning properly, which is hazardous. Bananas, oranges, and tomatoes are examples of foods high in potassium that patients with kidney failure may need to restrict their consumption of.

•**Phosphorus:** Patients with kidney failure may also suffer from bone and cardiac issues as a result of high phosphorus levels. Patients may need to restrict their use of phosphorus-rich foods like meat and dairy.

•**Fluids**: Kidney failure patients may need to restrict their fluid consumption to avoid fluid retention, which can lead to edema and high blood pressure.

Patients with renal failure may need to increase their intake of specific nutrients, such as protein, in addition to restricting certain foods and beverages. Protein is necessary for the growth and repair of tissues, however kidney failure patients may need to restrict their protein consumption to prevent further kidney damage. However, some individuals might need to consume more protein if they are receiving dialysis or have other illnesses that call for additional protein.

Patients with renal failure should collaborate closely with a qualified dietician with expertise in kidney disease in order to successfully manage their diet. A meal plan customized to the needs of each patient can be created with the dietitian's assistance, taking into account the patient's age, weight, general health, and personal preferences. The dietician can also offer advice on how to read food labels, make low-sodium and low-phosphorus meals, and choose healthy foods while dining out.

2. Organizing your Workout:

As it can help control weight, stress, and anxiety as well as enhance cardiovascular health, regular exercise is crucial for managing kidney failure. To prevent overexertion and injury, patients with renal failure might need to alter their exercise regimen. Before beginning an exercise program, patients should consult with their healthcare physician and adhere to the following rules:

•**Start slowly**: Patients should gradually increase the intensity and duration of their workouts, beginning with low-impact activities like walking or swimming.

•**Check blood pressure frequently**: Patients should monitor their blood pressure before and after exercise, and should stop if it rises too high.

•**Remain hydrated**: To avoid dehydration, patients should consume lots of fluids before to, during, and after exercise.

•**Avoid high-impact exercises**: Patients should refrain from sports like running or jumping that place a lot of stress on the joints.

In addition to adhering to these recommendations, patients should pay attention to their bodies and modify their workout regimen as necessary. Patients should avoid overexerting themselves and should stop working out if they feel pain, lightheaded, or out of breath.

3. Taking Care of Your Medications

In order to treat their symptoms and avoid complications, patients with renal failure may need to take drugs. It is crucial to remember that some medications can mix with other drugs and be detrimental to the kidneys. To make sure that their pharmaceutical regimen is secure and efficient, patients should consult with their doctor frequently.

A phosphate binder is one crucial drug that individuals with renal failure might need to take. These drugs aid in preventing the blood's phosphorus buildup, which can result in issues with the heart and bones. If a patient has diabetes, they may also need to take medicine to control their blood sugar levels, lower their cholesterol, and manage their high blood pressure.

Patients should take their drugs exactly as directed and contact their doctor if they have any side effects or difficulties taking their meds. Additionally, patients should refrain from taking dietary supplements or over-the-counter medicines without first talking to their doctor, as these might occasionally damage the kidneys.

Depression is a common mental health concern for patients with kidney failure. Symptoms of depression can include feelings of sadness, hopelessness, loss of interest in activities, and changes in appetite or sleep patterns. Depression can also cause physical symptoms such as fatigue, headaches, and digestive problems. Patients with depression may feel isolated and may have difficulty connecting with others, which can further exacerbate their symptoms.

Anxiety is another common mental health concern for patients with kidney failure. Anxiety can manifest in many different ways, such as feeling restless or on edge, having difficulty concentrating, and experiencing physical symptoms like sweating or a rapid heartbeat. Anxiety can also cause patients to avoid certain situations or activities, which can limit their quality of life.

Fear is another emotion that is common for patients with kidney failure. Fear can be related to the uncertainty of the future, concerns about the effectiveness of treatment, and worries about the impact of the illness on one's life and relationships. Fear can cause patients to feel overwhelmed and may make it difficult for them to take steps to manage their illness effectively.

It's important to address these mental health concerns because they can have a significant impact on a patient's overall well-being and quality of life. Untreated depression, anxiety, and fear can lead to a range of negative outcomes, including decreased ability to perform daily tasks, increased medical complications, and decreased treatment adherence.

One of the most effective ways to address mental health concerns is to seek professional help. Patients with kidney failure can benefit from working with a mental health professional such as a therapist, counselor, or psychologist. These professionals can provide support, guidance, and evidence-based treatments such as cognitive-behavioral therapy or medication. Mental health professionals can also help patients develop coping skills and strategies for managing their emotions and symptoms.

In addition to seeking professional help, there are many other steps that patients with kidney failure can take to improve their mental health. These include:

1. Building a support network: Patients with kidney failure should reach out to friends, family members, and support groups for emotional support. It can be helpful to talk to others who are going through similar experiences and who can offer advice, encouragement, and understanding.

2. Engaging in self-care activities: Self-care activities such as exercise, meditation, or hobbies can help patients manage their stress and improve their mood. Patients should try to incorporate these activities into their daily routine.

3.Prioritizing good sleep hygiene: Adequate sleep is essential for mental health. Patients with kidney failure should prioritize good sleep hygiene by establishing a regular sleep schedule, avoiding caffeine and alcohol before bedtime, and creating a comfortable sleep environment.

4.Maintaining a healthy lifestyle: A healthy lifestyle that includes a balanced diet, regular exercise, and avoiding smoking and excessive alcohol consumption can help improve both physical and mental health.

5. **Educating oneself about kidney failure**: Knowledge is power when it comes to managing kidney failure. Patients should educate themselves about their condition, including its symptoms, treatment options, and potential complications. This can help them feel more in control and empowered to manage their illness effectively.

6. **Communicating with healthcare providers**: Patients with kidney failure should communicate openly and honestly with their healthcare providers about their mental health concerns. Healthcare providers can provide support and guidance and can help connect patients with mental health resources.

In conclusion, addressing mental health concerns is essential for patients with kidney failure. Depression, anxiety, and fear can have a significant impact on a patient's overall well-being and quality of life. Patients should seek out professional help, build a support network, engage in self-care activities, prioritize good sleep hygiene, maintain a healthy lifestyle, educate themselves about kidney failure, and communicate openly with their healthcare providers. By taking these steps, patients can improve their mental health and better manage their illness, ultimately leading to a better quality of life.

Patients with renal failure may also benefit from other self-care activities like relaxation techniques, quitting smoking, and getting enough sleep in addition to these lifestyle changes. These procedures can enhance general health and wellbeing and assist patients in overcoming the mental and physical difficulties associated with renal failure.

In conclusion, altering one's lifestyle is a crucial component in managing kidney failure. Renal failure patients can successfully manage their condition by altering their diet, getting regular exercise, and taking their medications as directed. To make sure that their treatment plan is secure and efficient, patients should collaborate closely with their doctor and other medical experts like registered dietitians, fitness specialists, and pharmacists. Patients with kidney failure can enhance their general health and well-being, maintain a high quality of life, and take an active role in their care by changing their lifestyle.

The support network: Family, Friends and support groups

It can be difficult and intimidating to manage renal failure. It can be challenging to manage with the physical and psychological effects of the condition as well as the changes in your lifestyle. Patients with kidney failure can benefit greatly from having a solid support system. This network may consist of close relatives, close friends, medical professionals, and support organizations.

Patients with renal failure might benefit greatly from the emotional and practical assistance of family members and friends. They can lend a sympathetic ear, assist with everyday chores, and offer inspiration and motivation. Patients can be accompanied to appointments by family members and friends, who can also aid them with dietary changes and medication management. Being supported by family and friends can make patients feel less alone and give them a sense of comfort and security.

Patients with kidney failure might get help from healthcare professionals as well. These experts can offer counseling, emotional support, and both medical care and advice. Healthcare professionals can assist patients with managing their symptoms, understanding their treatment options, and addressing any worries or inquiries they may have. They can also recommend patients to other medical specialists who can offer more assistance and resources, such as social workers or mental health counselors.

A support group is another beneficial resource for many renal failure sufferers in addition to these other forms of assistance. Patients who are going through similar situations can connect with one another in a secure and encouraging environment provided through support groups. Healthcare professionals, as well as other patients and their families, may lead these gatherings. Support groups can convene in person or online and might concentrate on particular subjects like diet and nutrition, physical activity, or coping with the psychological effects of renal failure.

The advantages of joining a support group are numerous. Support groups, above all, foster a sense of belonging and community. Patients can talk about their feelings and experiences with those who can relate to them. Patients may feel less alienated and alone as a result, and they may also experience a sense of acceptance and affirmation. Support groups can also offer helpful pointers and recommendations for handling the difficulties of renal failure. Patients can obtain new ideas and views by reading about other people's experiences. Support groups can also give patients a private, secure setting in which to express their worries—something that can be challenging with family and friends.

Support groups can also provide people a sense of optimism and motivation, which is another advantage. The patient has the opportunity to interact with people who have successfully managed renal failure and gain knowledge from their experiences. Observing those who are thriving despite having renal failure can inspire and motivate patients and help them keep a good mindset.

Support groups for people with renal failure come in a wide variety of forms. While some groups are formal and organized by healthcare professionals or specialized organizations, others are informal and created by people. Patients might contact their healthcare practitioner for referrals or conduct an online search for local support groups. National organizations that provide resources and support for kidney disease patients include the National Kidney Foundation and the American Association of Kidney Patients.

It's critical to remember that support groups cannot replace medical treatment. Patients should keep in frequent contact with their doctor and adhere to their treatment regimen. Support groups, on the other hand, can be a beneficial addition to medical treatment and can give patients a sense of empowerment and control over their health.

In conclusion, managing with renal failure requires having a solid support system. Family, friends, medical professionals, and support organizations can all be helpful to patients with renal failure. These resources for help can offer both practical and emotional support, as well as a sense of belonging and community. Patients should use the many services at their disposal without holding back when asking for assistance. Patients with renal failure can enhance their general quality of life and attain improved health by cooperating with their support network.

Importance of mental health: overcoming fear, anxiety, and depression

Depression is a common mental health concern for patients with kidney failure. Symptoms of depression can include feelings of sadness, hopelessness, loss of interest in activities, and changes in appetite or sleep patterns. Depression can also cause physical symptoms such as fatigue, headaches, and digestive problems. Patients with depression may feel isolated and may have difficulty connecting with others, which can further exacerbate their symptoms.

Anxiety is another common mental health concern for patients with kidney failure. Anxiety can manifest in many different ways, such as feeling restless or on edge, having difficulty concentrating, and experiencing physical symptoms like sweating or a rapid heartbeat. Anxiety can also cause patients to avoid certain situations or activities, which can limit their quality of life.

Fear is another emotion that is common for patients with kidney failure. Fear can be related to the uncertainty of the future, concerns about the effectiveness of treatment, and worries about the impact of the illness on one's life and relationships. Fear can cause patients to feel overwhelmed and may make it difficult for them to take steps to manage their illness effectively.

It's important to address these mental health concerns because they can have a significant impact on a patient's overall well-being and quality of life. Untreated depression, anxiety, and fear can lead to a range of negative outcomes, including decreased ability to perform daily tasks, increased medical complications, and decreased treatment adherence.

One of the most effective ways to address mental health concerns is to seek professional help. Patients with kidney failure can benefit from working with a mental health professional such as a therapist, counselor, or psychologist. These professionals can provide support, guidance, and evidence-based treatments such as cognitive-behavioral therapy or medication. Mental health professionals can also help patients develop coping skills and strategies for managing their emotions and symptoms.

In addition to seeking professional help, there are many other steps that patients with kidney failure can take to improve their mental health. These include:

1. Building a support network: Patients with kidney failure should reach out to friends, family members, and support groups for emotional support. It can be helpful to talk to others who are going through similar experiences and who can offer advice, encouragement, and understanding.

2. Engaging in self-care activities: Self-care activities such as exercise, meditation, or hobbies can help patients manage their stress and improve their mood. Patients should try to incorporate these activities into their daily routine.

3.Prioritizing good sleep hygiene: Adequate sleep is essential for mental health. Patients with kidney failure should prioritize good sleep hygiene by establishing a regular sleep schedule, avoiding caffeine and alcohol before bedtime, and creating a comfortable sleep environment.

4.Maintaining a healthy lifestyle: A healthy lifestyle that includes a balanced diet, regular exercise, and avoiding smoking and excessive alcohol consumption can help improve both physical and mental health.

5. Educating oneself about kidney failure: Knowledge is power when it comes to managing kidney failure. Patients should educate themselves about their condition, including its symptoms, treatment options, and potential complications. This can help them feel

more in control and empowered to manage their illness effectively.

6. Communicating with healthcare providers: Patients with kidney failure should communicate openly and honestly with their healthcare providers about their mental health concerns. Healthcare providers can provide support and guidance and can help connect patients with mental health resources.

People with renal failure must be managed with a multifaceted strategy that may involve medication, treatment, and lifestyle modifications. Antidepressant drugs may occasionally be prescribed to treat the symptoms of depression. The symptoms of sadness and anxiety may also be managed with the aid of therapies like dialectical behavior therapy (DBT) and cognitive-behavioral therapy (CBT).

A nutritious diet, regular exercise, and stress-reduction methods like mindfulness and meditation can all assist to manage the symptoms of anxiety and depression. Exercise has been demonstrated to elevate mood and lessen signs of anxiety and despair. A balanced diet rich in fruits, vegetables, lean protein sources, and low in processed foods can also aid to enhance general mental wellness.

If you are experiencing renal failure-related mental health difficulties, it's crucial to seek expert assistance. Therapists, psychiatrists, and psychologists are just a few of the mental health specialists who may assist you in managing your symptoms and creating coping mechanisms that are effective for you.

It's critical to establish a solid support network in addition to getting expert assistance. During trying times, friends and family can offer moral support and encouragement. A sense of community and a connection with others who are going through comparable experiences can In conclusion, addressing mental health concerns is essential for patients with kidney failure. Depression, anxiety, and fear can have a significant impact on a patient's overall well-being and quality of life. Patients should seek out professional help, build a support network, engage in self-care activities, prioritize good sleep hygiene, maintain a healthy lifestyle, educate themselves about kidney failure, and communicate openly with their healthcare providers. By taking these steps, patients can improve their mental health and better manage their illness, ultimately leading to a better quality of life.

Patients with renal failure may also benefit from other self-care activities like relaxation techniques, quitting smoking, and getting enough sleep in addition to these lifestyle changes. These procedures can enhance general health and wellbeing and assist patients in overcoming the mental and physical difficulties associated with renal failure.

While managing the difficulties of renal failure might be challenging, it is possible to manage mental health problems and have a full life with the correct help and tools. It's critical to give
your mental health top priority and to get support if you need it. Despite the difficulties of renal failure, you can control your depressive and anxious symptoms with the correct care and carry on leading a fulfilling life.

CHAPTER 3:

HOPE AND INSPIRATION

Success stories: Real- life examples of individuals thriving with kidney failure

Being told that you have kidney failure can be terrifying, and it's easy to get caught up in the difficulties of treating this long-term condition. However, it's crucial to keep in mind that many people with renal failure are prospering and leading happy, successful lives. In this post, we'll give examples of people who have kidney failure and are thriving in real life and shed light on their success formulas.

1. Beth has had kidney failure for more than 20 years. Beth has been receiving dialysis ever since she received a kidney failure diagnosis more than 20 years ago. She has nevertheless managed to have a full and active life.

Her continued involvement in her community has been one of the factors in her success. Beth runs a knitting group at a community center where she volunteers and is active in her local church. She also likes to pursue her hobbies, go on walks in nature, and spend time with her family and friends.

Although Beth admits that having kidney failure presents some difficulties, she has managed the disease well. She prioritizes healthy eating, regular exercise, and good sleep hygiene. Additionally, she makes time for self-care pursuits like reading and meditation. Beth attributes her optimistic attitude on life to her faith and her adoring family and social network.

John: Doing well after a kidney transplant.
In his mid-thirties, John received a renal failure diagnosis; a few years later, he underwent a kidney transplant from a living donor. John has been doing well ever after the transplant and can now participate in many of the things he loved to do before his disease. He enjoys taking part in long charity rides as a passionate cyclist. John participates in his children's sports teams and takes his family on frequent family vacations.

John places a high focus on maintaining his physical fitness. He has a balanced diet, works out frequently, and takes his meds as directed. He also keeps in close contact with his medical professionals and schedules many follow-up visits to have his health checked. John is appreciative of the second chance at life that a kidney transplant has given him and realizes that it has changed his life.

3. Sarah: Fighting for both herself and those suffering from renal failure.

Midway through her twenties, Sarah received a kidney failure diagnosis and has been receiving dialysis ever since. She has discovered ways to use her illness for good by speaking out for kidney failure sufferers like herself. Sarah participates actively in her neighborhood support group and helps other patients as a peer mentor. She also takes part in advocacy campaigns to promote patient access to care and raise money for research into renal disease.

Although Sarah is aware that treating kidney failure might be difficult, she has found methods to remain upbeat and proactive. She prioritizes healthy eating, regular exercise, and proper sleep hygiene. She also does yoga and swimming. She also schedules time for self-care pursuits like reading and pet cuddling. Sarah attributes her support system and dedication to advocacy work for her accomplishment.

4. Michael: Discovering a new mission after developing renal failure

When Michael's kidney failure was discovered in his late 50s, he initially experienced depression and worry. He became a supporter of kidney disease research, nevertheless, after receiving his diagnosis, giving him a new sense of direction. Michael participates actively in a number of advocacy groups and has raised tens of thousands of dollars for scientific research. He urges others to take part in clinical trials and takes part himself.

Michael's ability to effectively manage his renal failure depends on maintaining a healthy lifestyle. He has a balanced diet, works out frequently, and takes his meds as directed. Additionally, he places a high priority on self-care pursuits like performing music, gardening, and spending time with loved ones. Michael attributes his success to his dedication to the cause of advocacy work as well as his network of devoted family and friends.

In conclusion, these actual cases show that people with kidney failure can thrive and have happy lives.

Advocacy and Awareness: Becoming an advocate for yourself and the community.

Being told you have renal failure might be frightening, but it can also be a chance to start speaking up for yourself and your neighborhood. Speaking out and acting on causes that are important to you is advocacy. Advocacy actions in the case of renal failure can aid in enhancing access to care, boosting research funding, and increasing public understanding of the condition. This article will examine the significance of advocacy and awareness for people with renal failure and will offer tips on how to be a successful advocate.

1. Recognizing the value of advocacy and education
For a number of reasons, advocacy and awareness are important for people with renal failure. First, advocacy

work can assist increase healthcare access. Financial, logistical, and geographical challenges can make it difficult for patients with renal failure to get the care they need. By supporting laws and plans that facilitate better access to healthcare, advocacy initiatives can assist in removing these obstacles.

Second, advocacy may enhance research funding. Kidney failure is a complicated and chronic ailment that necessitates continuous study to create novel cures and enhance results. Funding for research projects can be obtained through advocacy activities, which may result in innovations in the treatment of kidney failure.

For those who have renal failure, awareness is essential since it can lessen stigma and increase knowledge of the condition. Kidney failure is a problem that many people are unfamiliar with and may have misunderstandings about. Increased assistance for patients and their families as well as the promotion of accurate information regarding renal failure can all be a result of raising awareness.

2. Techniques for being a powerful advocate

You can become a successful advocate if you or a loved one has been diagnosed with renal failure by using a number of techniques.

•Educate yourself: Learning more about renal failure is the first step in being an effective advocate. Learn about the signs of kidney failure, the available treatments, and the difficulties that patients may encounter. Stay informed on the most recent advancements in kidney failure research and policy.

•Join a support group: For those with kidney failure, support groups may be a goldmine of knowledge and resources. They may also present chances to interact with other patients and exchange stories. Consider being a part of a local support group or online renal failure network.

•Participate in advocacy groups: There are a number of groups that support renal failure patients. Think about joining groups like the American Association of Kidney Patients or the National Kidney Foundation. These groups might offer chances to take part in advocacy activities and establish connections with other activists.

•Speak up: Being an advocate requires that you speak up and let others know about your experiences. Think about telling your tale to the media, your government leaders, or your local community. You can also take part in campaigns to raise awareness, such as kidney walks.

•Support policy change: Funding for research and access to care can both be significantly impacted by changes in policy. Consider promoting legislation that expand research funding, promote access to care, or lessen the impact renal failure has on patients and their families.

3. Case studies of effective advocacy initiatives

The care and results for people with renal failure have significantly improved as a result of advocacy activities. Here are a few instances of effective advocacy work:

•The National renal Foundation successfully lobbied for the Medicare ESRD program, which covers dialysis and transplantation for qualified patients, to cover renal disease.

•The Living Donor Protection Act, which shields living organ donors from discrimination in insurance and employment, was passed thanks to the strong advocacy work of the American Association of Kidney Patients.

•The Patient Ambassador Program was introduced by the Renal Support Network, which educates and empowers patients and their families to become champions for kidney disease awareness.

•The Kidney Precision Medicine Project, a research initiative aimed at creating new treatments for kidney illness, was started by the National Institute of Diabetes and Digestive and Kidney Diseases (NIDDK).

4. Guidelines for effective advocacy

Although advocating for yourself and your community can be difficult, there are a few strategies that can help.

• Be ready: Make sure you are ready before you speak up or take action. Study the topic you are arguing for, compile pertinent facts and figures, and hone your argument.

•Focus on solutions: When arguing for a cause, it's critical to highlight solutions rather than issues. Identify particular laws or initiatives that could ease access to care, boost research funding, or lessen stigma.

•Create relationships: You may further your advocacy efforts by creating connections with other activists, healthcare professionals, and lawmakers. Participate in gatherings and events, network with others, and work together on advocacy projects.

•Be persistent: Although advocating can be a drawn-out and difficult process, persistence is essential. Even though change is being made slowly, keep speaking up and acting.

•enjoy achievements: When advocacy efforts yield fruitful results, take some time to recognize and enjoy those achievements. This may increase momentum and motivate further participants.

In conclusion, support and education are essential for those with kidney failure. Increased financing for research, better access to care, and a reduction in stigma are all benefits of advocacy work. There are several ways to become a successful advocate, including educating yourself, finding a support group, getting involved with advocacy groups, speaking out, and pushing for legislative change. Kidney failure sufferers can improve their own lives as well as the lives of others by acting and speaking out.

The future of research and treatment for kidney failure

Millions of individuals throughout the world suffer from the dangerous condition of kidney failure. While there is still a tremendous need for better therapies and a cure, treatment methods including dialysis and transplantation have improved throughout time. We will examine the current state of renal failure treatment and research in this article, as well as the optimistic advancements that lie ahead.

•Present Treatment Alternatives

Dialysis and transplantation are the two main kidney failure treatments. When the kidneys are unable to filter waste from the blood on their own, a method called dialysis is used to do so. Hemodialysis and peritoneal dialysis are the two forms of dialysis. While peritoneal dialysis uses the lining of the abdominal cavity to filter the blood, hemodialysis uses a machine that filters the blood outside of the body.

A healthy kidney from a donor is used to replace the damaged kidney during transplantation. Living or deceased donors can both provide kidneys. Living donation is favored since it provides better results and shortens the transplant waiting period.

Medications to regulate blood pressure and treat symptoms, as well as dietary and activity changes, are other treatments for renal failure.

•Problems with Current Therapy

Even though dialysis and transplantation have significantly elevated the quality of life for many renal failing patients, they are not without drawbacks. Dialysis is time-consuming, and patients may have negative side effects like exhaustion, low blood pressure, and cramping. Due to a lack of organ donors, transplantation is not always possible, and even when it is, the recipient must take immunosuppressant drugs for the rest of their lives to prevent rejection of the new kidney.

The underlying causes of kidney failure, which can include a number of conditions like diabetes, hypertension, and hereditary diseases, are not currently addressed by available treatments. More specialized treatments are required to stop or delay the course of renal disease.

•Regenerative Medicine's Promise

Regenerative medicine is one of the most exciting fields of study for treating renal failure. In this method, damaged kidney tissue is repaired or replaced utilizing stem cells or other cell-based therapies. Both adult stem cells and induced pluripotent stem cells (iPSCs), which can be produced from a patient's own skin cells, are being investigated by researchers.

Cell-based therapies for renal illness are currently being put through a number of clinical trials to determine their safety and effectiveness. The Kidney Project is one such trial, with the goal of creating an implanted bioartificial kidney that can perform like a healthy kidney. The device is now undergoing preclinical testing and is being created utilizing human kidney cells and nanotechnology.

The application of gene therapy to the treatment of renal disease is a potential new field of study. To fix genetic abnormalities that lead to kidney failure, researchers are looking at using gene editing methods like CRISPR.

•Personalized Care and Precision Medicine

Precision medicine is a method of providing healthcare that involves customizing treatments for each patient based on their specific traits, such as

genetics, environment, and lifestyle. As it can assist identify individuals who are at risk for renal failure and customize treatment to meet those needs, this strategy has considerable potential for the treatment of kidney disease.

To enhance precision medicine in the field of renal disease, several initiatives are now under way. The Kidney Precision Medicine Project, spearheaded by the National Institute of Diabetes and Digestive and Kidney Diseases (NIDDK), intends to find novel therapeutic targets and provide innovative kidney disease diagnostic tools.

•The Treatment of Kidney Failure in the Future

The therapy of renal failure has a bright future ahead of it, with numerous encouraging advancements in the works. A better quality of life for those with kidney failure is possible because to current research in regenerative medicine, gene therapy, and precision medicine.

Regenerative medicine is a promising field of study for the treatment of renal failure. By utilizing stem cells, fresh kidney tissue can be grown, possibly replacing sick or damaged kidneys. Regenerative medicine has demonstrated encouraging results in animal studies and clinical trials while being in its early phases of development.

The creation of wearable and transportable artificial kidneys, which would offer a more practical and comfortable substitute to conventional dialysis, is another topic of research. The patient wears or carries these devices, which enable continuous, on-the-go dialysis therapy.

The use of immunosuppressant drugs to slow the progression of kidney damage in specific conditions and the use of genetic testing to identify people who may be at risk for developing kidney disease are two additional approaches that researchers are looking into.

Overall, with ongoing technological and medical improvements, the future of renal failure therapy and research is positive. Although managing renal failure and improving quality of life can be difficult for people, there are numerous tools available to support them. We can work toward a time when kidney failure is no longer a potentially fatal condition through activism, support systems, and medical innovation.

CONCLUSION

Embracing Hope: living your best life with kidney failure

Although living with renal failure can be difficult, it is still possible to embrace hope and lead a happy life.

Here are some pointers for thriving despite kidney failure:

•Remain Positive: When dealing with renal failure, a positive outlook can go a long way. Spend time with positive individuals and pay attention to the things that make you happy and fulfilled in life. Keep your hobbies and aspirations in mind, but don't allow your illness define you or prevent you from pursuing them.

•Remain Active: Physical activity and exercise can help control the signs and symptoms of renal failure as well as your general health and wellbeing. Consult your doctor about the best forms of exercise for your particular situation.

•Manage Your Diet: Dietary management is essential for treating renal failure. Create a salt-, potassium-, and phosphorus-free healthy eating plan in collaboration with a trained nutritionist. Your entire health will benefit and your kidneys' stress will be lessened as a result.

•Manage Your Medications: It's crucial to take your medications as directed and to let your healthcare team know if you have any questions or experience any negative effects. Keep a note of your prescriptions and their recommended dosages, and bring it to every doctor's appointment.

•Seek Support: Getting in touch with individuals who are dealing with renal failure or joining a support group can make you feel less alone and offer insightful guidance. It's crucial to express your demands and worries to your loved ones as well as the medical staff.

•Pay attention to self-care: Maintaining your mental health and general wellbeing is essential if you have renal failure. Engage in self-care practices like yoga, deep breathing, or meditation. Take part in pastimes and activities that make you happy and relieve stress.

•Take Charge of Your Health: Participate actively in your treatment and healthcare. Learn about your disease and available treatments, and when necessary, speak up for yourself. With your medical team, express your needs and concerns and ask questions.

Living a full and meaningful life despite having kidney failure is achievable if you embrace hope and take charge of your health and wellbeing. Always keep the big picture in mind and concentrate on the good things in your life. Anything is achievable if you have the correct attitude and support.

Lasting Thoughts and Encouragement

Although managing renal failure might be difficult, it's crucial to keep in mind that you are not alone. To assist you manage your health and lead the best possible life, there are tools and support services available. Here are a few last words of wisdom and motivation to get you through this journey:

Living with kidney failure can be overwhelming, but it's crucial to keep your attention on the here and now and take each day as it comes. Don't be too hard on yourself when things don't go according to plan, and instead, celebrate your accomplishments and minor achievements.

•Exercise self-compassion: When coping with renal failure, it's crucial to be nice to yourself and exercise self-compassion. This entails treating oneself with the same compassion and consideration that you would show a dear friend or family member.

•Remain informed: Become knowledgeable about your condition and keep up with new developments in both treatment and research. This can aid in your decision-making regarding your health and course of treatment.

•Create a support system: Get in touch with people who are also dealing with kidney failure, whether through support groups, online forums, or real-world gatherings. This can make you feel less alone and offer insightful guidance.

•Hold onto hope: Even with renal failure, it is still possible to have a full and meaningful life. Focus on the good things in your life, such as spending time with family and friends, following your passions, or attaining your goals.

•Ask for assistance when you need it; don't be ashamed to do so. When aid is required, get in touch with your support network, loved ones, or medical team.

• Speak out for yourself: Take an active role in your treatment and healthcare. Speak up for yourself and let your healthcare staff know what you need and are worried about. You have a right to information and to participation in your care.

Despite the difficulties that may come with having renal failure, it is still possible to live a happy life. Keep in mind to look after yourself, be informed, and get support.

Accept hope, and concentrate on the good things in your life. Anything is achievable if you have the correct attitude and support.

It's crucial to keep in mind that, despite the potential for life-altering consequences, renal failure is not a fatal diagnosis. Many people with renal failure have successfully completed this journey and are now leading happy lives. You may manage your illness and yet follow your interests and objectives.

Keeping a positive outlook is one of the keys to leading a good life despite kidney failure. This does not imply disregarding the difficulties brought on by the disease; rather, it means learning how to manage them and putting your attention on the good things in your life. Finding enjoyable pursuits such as spending time with loved ones, partaking in hobbies, or exploring new interests may be necessary to achieve this.

Maintaining a healthy lifestyle is crucial for people who have kidney failure. This may entail eating kidney-friendly foods, exercising frequently, and taking any recommended medications as indicated. To create a treatment plan that is customized for you, it is crucial to engage closely with your medical team.

Prioritizing your mental health is equally as vital as prioritizing your physical health. Having measures in place to control these emotions is crucial since living with renal failure may be stressful and anxiety-inducing. This can entail speaking with a therapist, joining a group, or practicing relaxation methods like yoga or meditation.

Being your own best advocate when it comes to your medical care and treatment plan is also crucial. This entails raising issues, voicing your worries, and speaking up for the services and resources you require in order to properly manage your disease. Always keep in mind that you are a vital part of your healthcare team and have the right to information and involvement in your treatment.

Finally, it's critical to understand that, despite the difficulties of living with renal failure, there are also chances for growth and personal development. Many people who have made it through this journey have reported feeling more resilient, thankful, and compassionate toward others. You may overcome the difficulties of renal failure and live your best life by embracing hope and concentrating on the good facets of your life.

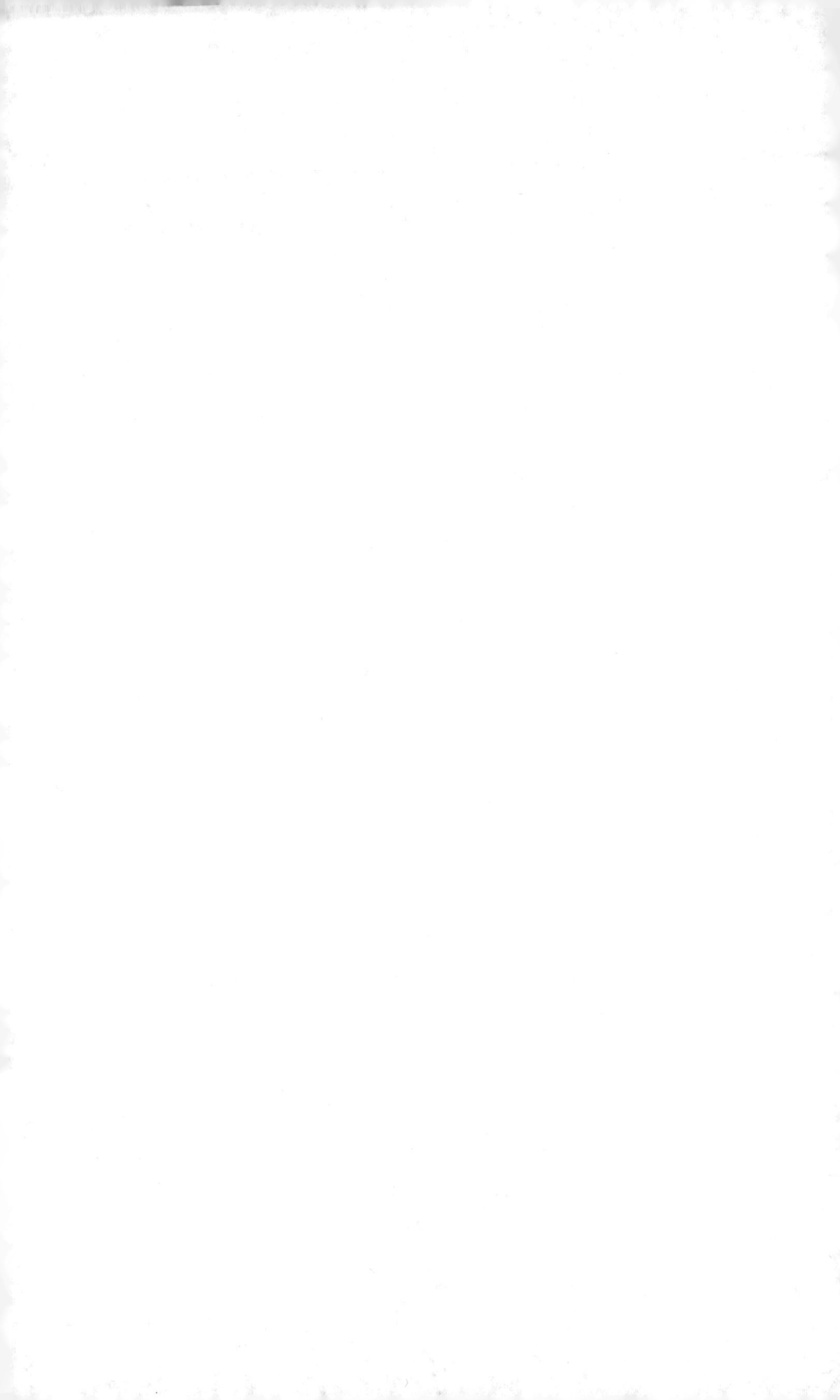